ANTIEMETIC FOR HOMESICKNESS

ANTIEMETIC FOR HOMESICKNESS

Romalyn Ante

Chatto & Windus
LONDON

1 3 5 7 9 10 8 6 4 2

Chatto & Windus, an imprint of Vintage,
20 Vauxhall Bridge Road,
London SW1V 2SA

Chatto & Windus is part of the Penguin Random House group of companies
whose addresses can be found at global.penguinrandomhouse.com

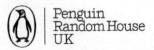

First published by Chatto & Windus in 2020

penguin.co.uk/vintage

A CIP catalogue record for this book is available from the British Library

ISBN 9781784743000

Typeset in 11/14 pt Minion Pro
by Integra Software Services Pvt. Ltd, Pondicherry

Printed and bound in Great Britain by Clays Ltd, Elcograf S.p.A.

Penguin Random House is committed to a sustainable future for our business,
our readers and our planet. This book is made from Forest Stewardship
Council® certified paper.

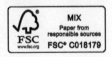

for my mother

*Love your solitude, accept the pain it causes you,
and make a melody with it.*

– RAINER MARIA RILKE

Contents

Half-empty 1

Names 3

The Making of a Smuggler 6

Patis 8

Way Back Home 9

Mateo 11

Notes inside a Balikbayan Box 12

Tape Recordings for Mama 14

To Die a Little 16

#family 18

Anagolay 19

Lanzones 20

At the Other End of the Bridge 21

Tagay! [Drinking Lambanog with my Filipino Colleagues] 22

Nature Morte aux Tulipes 27

Invisible Women 28

[   ] 30

ꪩꪀꪮꪶ 36

Eponym 38

The Shaman, The Servant 39

Repairing English 43

Mastering English 44

Anosmia 45

Only Distance 46

The Wait 47

Checkmate 50

Respecting the Nunò 52

For the Dance Festival 53

A Manananggal Replies to a Child 55

relearning 58

Kayumanggi 59

Ode to a Pot Noodle 60

Group Portrait at the Stopover 61
Para sa mga batang naiwan
  or For the children left behind 63
Antiemetic for Homesickness 64

A Boodle Fight of Words and Terminologies 67
Notes 70
Acknowledgements 73

x

ANTIEMETIC FOR HOMESICKNESS

Half-empty

'The Philippines must be half-empty; you're all here running the NHS.' – PRINCE PHILIP, DUKE OF EDINBURGH

Drug:
Migrationazoline (available in full or half-empty bottles)

Indications:
- prophylaxis of parents who nag like surgical drills
  saying they did not send you to college
  to become a healthcare volunteer
- episodic blindness secondary to power cuts
- ulcers on the lips from eating *kamote* or *kangkong* every night
- chronic ache for a house and garden of your own
- chest tightness and/or dyspnoea as you watch your child
  drool over Special Siomai

Contraindications:
- do not take this medicine if you have a weak stomach
  or sensitivity to the tug of your child at your skirt

Cautions:
- your husband may look for another lover while you're gone
- you may not be able to fly back home in time
  for your mother's burial
- your child may forget your name

Side effects:
- drowsiness/vertigo/nausea
- behavioural changes
- weight loss (when you deprive yourself of a steak bake
  and ceaselessly convert pounds to peso)
- severe acne (unknown relatives who demand money)

- low mood (on occasions as *Noche Buena*)
- bloating (as you yearn for the sweetness of *lanzones*
  or see flakes of desiccated coconut in the black November sky)
- intermittent euphoria (when you hand the bald girl
  her crocheted unicorn hat and her mother the discharge form)
- acute insomnia (when a child on a stretcher is rushed
  through the door – his face blood-soaked, and for a second
  you think of the one you left back home)

Names

'We are nameless, and all names are ours.'
– EMMANUEL LACABA

My mother's name is Rosana, but when she left,
I had other mothers. Rowena, Jimboy, Alma.

      I was named after
      the first syllables of my parents;
      I will always have them with me.

My mother says not all names have meaning –
Riverside. Manila. London. Kurba.

      And someday I will forget
      all the commands I did not heed –
like the time I did not spin the plate clockwise
      before my father left for work
even if it would deliver him from accidents.

Not all destinations are found
in the junctions of your palm lines.
Say better life, say better life.

      And God knows I am repenting.

Say airbus-something, say one-way ticket,
keep following the sunset.   Clouds
are the closest things to my mother.

Say United Kingdom, say the queen, NHS.
Does winter always mean —   ?

Listen – can you hear it? The loneliness
of stretchers along A&E corridors.

And the strongest part of me
is the scar I hide underneath my fringe.

My mother
hides in the staff toilet
to make long-distance calls.

Someday I will realise
the woman lonely in her mansion
is not my mother
but a future version of myself.
I will chop bitter gourds
on the galaxy-glimmer
of her worktop.

Shall we shorten your name on your nametag
so it's easier to remember? Say Yes please, Sister.

Say Please, Sister, can I take this call?

Say Arnold, Marcus, Harold. Say septicaemia, alcohol
poisoning, hernia.
Say Jason, Darius, Vernon. Say cancer, myocardial
infarction, query schizophrenia.

Hides in the toilet.

And I have the first syllables
of my parents' names,
that is why I am not scared.

4

A boy sticks out his tongue
and says I do not have a mother.
I punch him in the face. The sanctity of blood.

I am not scared.

Because my mother has followed the sunset,
because she has burnt her lips on mash and gravy
in a three-minute lunch break.
Because she calls me *Anak* – my child, my baby.
She asks, What do you want for Christmas? for your
birthday?

1990 remains stuck on the other line.
Say Please, Sister, can I take this call?

My breasts blossom,
she can call me only by my name.

I have the first syllables of my parents' names,
that is why I am not scared.

I can trek the mountain of Makulot,
my father's rifle hanging from my back.

I can carry myself
not how someone carries
a cytotoxic drug
but how my mother hooks
with her finger, a drain bottle
with blood clots the weight
of gemstones.

The Making of a Smuggler

Wherever we travel, we carry
the whole country with us –

our rice terraces are folded garments,
we have pillars of trees, a rainforest

on a hairbrush. We dig *alimasag* crabs
out of sand and use them as tabs

to zip our bags. We immigrants
are experts in packing. It's in our genes.

If the Border Officer stops us,
let him dive into our belongings

like a man trying to fish in an ocean
ruled by sharp corals, stinging anemones.

Let the smell of old socks swirl up like bats.
He can squeeze the yellow packet harder

and not know it is pig's blood. He won't
hear the squeal as he chucks it aside –

he wasn't there, mud-soaked in a pen,
chasing after the erratic swine.

The officer might ask, *No sauce?*
No chicken feet? with a broken accent

as if it would be easier for us to understand
but he can't smell my hands, see the sediments

under my nails – fermented fish and all
we dip in it. He can't cup his ear

with my palm and hear the surfs
of Siargao beach. He can't follow me

through the gate, even with his gaze.
He'll miss the gleam of a red quill

in my lug sole, as when he didn't hear
my uncle's knife grind back and forth

on a whetstone, or how he slit the neck
of my rooster to teach me about survival.

The officer did not feel the pot
of hot water getting lighter

when I poured it over the carcass.
He wasn't there, at that moment –

where I ripped out the feathers
I once used to caress.

Patis

There is a certain sour-salt taste
I always long for: sheen pieces of bullet tuna
wrapped in banana leaves, with sun-dried
kamias, simmered in a terracotta pot.

My grandma's specialty, moist to the bone,
best eaten with boiled rice and bare hands.
Two decades on, no one cooks *patis* anymore.
My grandma, in her wheelchair, calls me 'sister'.

The locals no longer nap in the grotto
of bougainvillea. The paddy fields
now a steadfast highway.
There is a Batangas I cannot return to –

gathered round my grandma's table
glazed by dusk, where each of us
takes a pinch of the rich fish flesh
and all we need is in our reach.

Way Back Home

'The way home is a thousand leagues.' – YI YANG-YON

Whenever you are lost,
my father told me,
you must turn your shirt inside out.

> As a family, we reversed
> our tropical print vests
> when instead of white sands
> we found a barren land
> of black stones,
> wrecked plastic bottles
> like a smack of jellyfish.

In childhood, when my siblings
left me by the rice sack swing,
I flipped my blouse and found
my heart became a ripe *makopa*
with ants instead of seeds at the core.

> I followed my father's advice
> and survived the hypnotic gaze
> of a *pavo*, and the buffalo
> that stood as a gatekeeper
> between me and my way home.

I found the landmark:
the chapel
where my father confessed
his feelings for my mother,
where scents of *sampaguita*
emanated from Christ's stigmata.

Now in a foreign land
all the red buses are stranded –
I stroll in ankle-deep snow
back to the flat with hallway walls
that rustle with my parents'
divorce papers.

In the lamp-lit flurry
I stop to take my coat off
and turn it inside out.

Mateo

'Look at the birds of the air, for they neither sow nor reap nor gather into barns.'—MATTHEW, 6:26

But birds have no bills.
So, she flew to a country where
the winds were feathers and talons,
scraping the iced   asphalt,
where the noon sky   blackened
and the carers by
day became experts
of drinking games
by night, where
the wallpaper warmed as a bag of blood
and the bloke brought in by an ambulance
borrowed her father's name, whose whist-
ling stopped-and-
started at a memory
he briefly grasped
then lost. It was that
call: when her father
said he got the money.   It was the weight
of light through the   venetian blinds, her
dappled cheek that echoed   the refrain of gold-
finches. It was the remembering – that morning
she saw her boy walking unshod, baptising his ankles
in the mud – a pair of shoes in his hand, one with
a peeling sole. It was that dazzling life, the piggy-
back, the kisses behind her ear.

Notes inside a Balikbayan Box

Dear son,
In my place, here is a Balikbayan box.
Here are the LeBron James rubber shoes (size 9)
and the video game tapes to replace all the palm cakes
I owe you for every *Simbang Gabi* and PTA meeting
I could not attend. I promise I'll be there for Christmas.
I know I've been saying this for a decade now.

Find the E45 cream for your grandma's tissue-dry skin,
a stack of incontinence pads and tubes of barrier balm.
Between you and me: every time I roll old people
onto their sides and lift their knees to their chests
for suppositories, I ask myself, *Who does this for her?*

Tell Tita to leave her husband. Her *school sweetheart*
whose mistresses are *mah-jong* and *sabong.* Tell her
not to bear the stink of his armpits. In the box
find the Gucci Bloom perfume and scar creams. Tell her
I haven't forgotten our vows when we were young
and our fingers smelled of *li hing mui* candies.
Our *Walang Iwanan* oath to never leave each other.

Dear son,
In my place, here is a Balikbayan Box.
Rip all the packaging tape – every gift inside is yours.
Work your hands hard until there's nothing left.
Learn that to survive we must have strong arms.
To carry a tray full of medicine and not let one
drop, to push a hyperventilating woman (with speed
and care) to the Maternity Wing, to lift and sit
a skin-and-bone man down on his chemo chair,

to gauge the weight of a rose before you lay it
onto a coffin. Take this box inside our house –
that is all I ask you to carry, for now, my son.

Ma, *kamusta na?*
Is it true? London Bridge
is huge enough to hold
the weight of our village?

Outside San Sebastian church
a homeless family
shares *taro* leaves in a can.
Ma, I finally understand –

they're hungry but complete,
ourselves full but fractured.
You taught me: to be blessed
is to bleed.

Tape Recordings for Mama

Ma, today in the woods
I found a young *haribon*
jammed its head into a tree hole.
Darkness could not make it flinch.

Today my classmates pointed at a map
of blood on the back of my skirt.
One said it was *United Kingdom.*
Laughter could not make me flinch.

———————————————

Tape Recordings for Mama

To Die a Little

'Partir es un poco morir, llegar nunca es llegar...' – ORACION DE MIGRANTES

'When I left you, I had to kill a part of my heart.' – MAMA

You stood on the other side of the barrier,
time is a tattered blanket draped down your shoulders.

My tympanic membrane beat what you held back,
Ma, wag mo akong iwan. Ma, don't leave me.

Our day clattered down the litter, a snail-slow plane
cut across our sky. I learned the routine: drawing a cross

on each day of the calendar. In and out, in and out
of the automatic-door mouth of a concrete god.

There, in the unchecked wound of the world, you lie on a bed,
IV drips hang over your head like a battery-drained cot toy.

Here, I set a vomit bowl under someone else's chin
and watch him sleep as the walls convulse in magma-hot breaths.

Here's the truth: my tympanic membrane beats,
wala kang kwenta, useless mother.

*

You said all I needed to do was to sleep and before I knew it,
you'd be back. But I woke to the rice that needed rinsing,
my siblings' school uniforms that needed ironing.

I woke to a refrain of drunkards across the road.
A man in a cowboy hat plucked his *gitara*

and sang about the woman who packed a suitcase,
> *Just when I needed you most.*

I woke when the washing machine broke
and beat clothes at the backyard.
A sleepy face frothing in a puddle,
> *Just when I needed you most.*

I raised my head above the waves
of smoke from a burning wok and wondered
if the swirl of black mist would reach you.

But I believed, Mama – before I knew it, you'd be back.
When I yanked my sister by her hair for answering back,
I held on to what you said.

When I choked on phlegm at midnight,
missing the ginger-kick of your *tinola*,
I held on to what you said.

When other mothers climbed to the stage
to pin medals to my classmate's chests,
I held on to what you said.

On Sundays, I played *tumbang preso* with the other kids.
We laughed because we were not orphans, only left behinds.
A swift hit – a rubber flip-flop knocked down an empty can

and the years clanked down the street. The smell of rain
lifted the dust from the road as I sprinted for a shelter,
> *Just when I needed you most.*

#family

This whole time I'd been reading it wrong,
seeing only broken things.
In Orthopaedics, # is read as 'fracture' –
#NoF is 'fractured neck of femur',
#collarbone is 'fractured collarbone'.

When I was young, my mother dabbed
dalanghita oil onto her hands, to soothe
a fissure in my chest – a finger swept
the muscle between my ribs. The window
trembled with fractures of lightning
as frayed shadows swallowed the room.
I focused on her touch and everything
eased into the fluster of leaves.

But I woke to the clatter of her luggage
to find her gone.
Perhaps that is how every waking hour begins.
Now I rub Vicks on my breastbone, hoping
the storm beneath will cease. I tread a dislocated
world, and each spot I step onto cleaves.

Anagolay

I do not ask for divine reappearance.
Let the misplaced objects recede in the heat
of an isolated island – where sunlight
snakes across the underwater sand.
Let the lost things grain the night sky
against the blurred edges of Milky Way.
I had travelled so far I could no longer hear
the waves heaving onto a shore accessible only
through below the towers of limestone rocks,
where a gap closes like a promise at high tide.
Anagolay, help me find a torch-pen in the peril
of a drug trolley. Help me retrieve the will
of my patient who pushes all pills aside,
with the back of a hand. Guide me, for I have
walked against the wind that is always homeward,
for I return to find my own children tread past me
as if I were a palm tree thrashed by thunderstorms.
Goddess of lost things, today a space council
names an asteroid after you, and tonight,
another world ebbs, a punctured lung.
A torch ticks on – its beam leads to my children's
sand-speckled feet. Let me look up to remember
the fifth vital sign has always been pain.
Let me find a prick of light gliding like a plane
or if not, the rhythm of a shockable heart.

Lanzones

Once, you brought me a bouquet
of *lanzones*. A yellow lump
thumbed open. Under our tree,
all brilliance swayed.

You were always a know-it-all –
burning dried rinds at my father's yard,
saying the smoke repelled mosquitoes
and anything that crawled.

The news came from your uncle
and our tree thumped all night.
Do you remember my breath
cooling your knuckles

daubed with Betadine?
You convinced me to go, lying
about England: *It's a brighter place.*
Pagka-daming lamok dine.

But memory continues to burn
like yesterday's mosquito bite.
For two years you'd picked
overripe fruits thrown

by summer, until one night
they found you on a rooftop –
sipping sugarcane wine,
hurling *lanzones* seeds

at a distance they could never reach.

At the Other End of the Bridge

They cannot recall the explosion
of wings the day he watched her
walk the length of the bridge.

Gone are the nights he steals
the moon with a mango picker
and swaps it for her pocket mirror

and gone are the days she harvests
scales from the claws of an eagle
and uses them to bind his scars.

Tagay! [Drinking Lambanog with my Filipino Colleagues]

It's my turn, *Tagay!*
This 80 proof our talisman for survival.
One day, we'll go home, I'll go home
and scan the crowd for the smile
that opens only to me at Arrivals.

It's my turn, *Tagay!*
The window is pockmarked by hailstones
but someday, Manila's heat will smother us
and thaw our frosted lungs –

my veins will throb in the orchestra
of jeepneys –

the road quivers in their silver shimmer.
I'll hop on and hunch along the aisle to sit
in the sliver of gap between passengers,
their sweat-slicked arms fused to mine.

It's my turn, *Tagay!*
When I get home my bag will burst
with Toblerone and Cadbury –
my children will lick the melted years
off their palms as they listen to my story
of the giant of Mount Montalban
who shakes his leg to make earthquakes.
But at night my wife and I are certain –
true belonging is where curtains unfasten
and a kiss clicks like a bedside lamp,

where earthquakes happen on top
or underneath our bed linen.

Now it's my turn, *Tagay!*
I imagine each day as a *Dating gawi* –
just like the old times.

Tito and I will flag down a tricycle,
judder over potholes, inhale the town's
exhaust on the way to Lipa's Panciteria.

Bowls of *lomi* will thump in front of us,
its soup thickened with cassava flour –
the meat-chunk odour of *miki* noodles

oozes through crammed toppings
of liver slices and pork scratchings.
Until then, *Tagay!*

It's my turn –
light shatters in the dregs of this bottle.
Tomorrow we'll be changing bed covers,
soaking dentures, creaming cracked heels
but before I know it
                    I'll be with my brother
driving to San Juan –
along the larimar gloss of the ocean.
Our skin brined and burnt – we'll feel the jerk
of curved palmyra trunks
                    as we backflip and splatter

into clear waters. We'll lie in a rainbow
hammock, drowsy in the clatter
of *capiz* shell windchimes.

It's my turn, *Tagay!*
In this flat, we stink like *sardinas.*
Soon I'll trace the nut-sweet hint
of *pan de coco* in a woven canister
on the back of a pedlar's bicycle.
Ka Celie will call from the corner,
Kelan ka dumating? When did you return?
She's as young as the day I left –
still pegging *tinapa* fish on the laundry line.

When the midday sun sears my nape
my school mates and I will congregate
on the terrace – passing around a karaoke mic
and a chaser of coconut wine.

As the alcohol knocks everyone out
like the summer that pummelled Pacquiao,
I will saunter with my childhood crush
in my *Lolo*'s orchard –
under the chandelier of jade vines.

This last shot is mine, *Tagay!*
I've just arrived, and autumn
has already settled in my eyes.
I'll get used to the English cold –
each time I push a plunger
I'll find, in the needle-tip bead,
a mangrove lagoon.
If I endure, I'll earn enough
for Papa's heart operation.

Here's to you, *Tagay!*
Soon, a morning will explode
into the camphor-fume of birds' droppings
in a basement that beats with eighty
thousand *balinsasayaw*. I'll harvest
their dense saliva-nests on the ceiling
and tweezer out the stuck feathers
before boiling them in chicken stock.
It would be just like the old times –

Papa and I will slurp bowls of nest soup
as we sit on cracked, upturned pots
amongst the haematoma of flowers.

Until then, I'll wear double-double layers.
Until then, *Tagay!*

Ma, it is *Semana Santa*. The townsmen
are pelting their backs with stingray tails.
Flesh slashes open, broils with sinful blood.
Their ears sear in April light, their foreheads
dotted with clots from thorn-crown stabs.

Ka Putol lays down on the road, opens
his palms to the luminosity of clouds.
Tonight, he sits under our jackfruit tree
and stares beyond his bandaged hands –
he tells me a body is an endless penitence.

How much longer must we wait, Ma?

––––––––––––––––––––––––––––––––––––

Tape Recordings for Mama

Nature Morte aux Tulipes

Oil paint on canvas, 1932

They can take her out of the freezer
but no one can thaw her skull, her shinbone.
The ligaments and tendons cannot be sewn again –
bone to tissue, bone to bone. No one will ever see
how the scars on her arm resemble the shapes
of Islas de Gigantes, her province's paradise.
She will never hear the keening of a grounded bird's
engine, the hands throbbing on the casket, *their* words.
She cannot inhale, again, the musk of roasted rice,
complete the half-built hut in the field, or escape
to the corner of a soil once shaded by the avocado tree
before the tug of monsoon. Sometimes rain
sings only to itself. No one can glue her bones
back in place. No one can learn her laughter.

Invisible Women

You see them everywhere, these invisible women –
    one navigates the ache of a corridor and the hour glints
    with a salvo of needles. A steel intubating stylet
    enters a mouth like a forced prayer.

On the news, an invisible woman fell asleep
    on the steering wheel and somersaulted into daybreak –
    debris glittering across the motorway.

A splinter buries deeper – she speaks to her patient
    about his petunias but doesn't mention the blooms
    of tumours on his endoscopy scan.

They are everywhere, though some hazier than others.
    Flick through their passports to find only a page –
    their names and countries erased by sun rays.

These invisible women, goddesses of caring and tending,
    but no one hears when their skulls pound
    like coconut shells about to crack.

My mother walks to work when the sky is black
    and comes out from work when the sky is black,
    her footsteps leave a snowdrop-studded path.

In the middle of a plaza, she pauses –
    the downpour tricking her eyes to believe
    the statue in the square is a fellow invisible woman.

Once, my mother cut through the blurred backs of men
       towards a gasping child, and found
    a blade of grass fluttering in his throat.
    The air opened and she was gone.

[   ]

1.

Already I am on a bus.
It is snowing horizontally.
The bus careens and propels me
into a snowball that splatters

on someone's chest.

Already I am in the blur
of a treatment cubicle,
handing the doctor a blade
to slit the throat of a man
who asphyxiates
in his own *lahar* of vomit.

A food tray on a table,
a woman with potash perm
gapes at the steam of roast potatoes –
she clangs the metal lid down.

Lights out.

2.

Many monsoons ago
a *sepulturero* looked up at us
and asked where to rebury the bones.

But before bones were just bones
they were my Nanay Lola,

a woman lolling in a night so quiet
you could hear the shallow
diastole of stars.

3.
San ibabaon ito?
Where do I bury the bones?
The *sepulturero*'s voice
thick like loam before a storm.

4.
Stifled
by surgical-bright lights
the miasma of antiseptic   and Hibiscrub
                    footsteps smack

the swish-snap
        of plastic aprons   slap of latex gloves

            cardiac monitors
                    bleep bleep
                bleep bleepbleep
                    bleep_____

5.
This is a place where you can master
selective hearing –
the machines
versus
the impatient patient
who criticises even a cup of tea,

the flashes of an ambulance
versus

the thoughts of an old man
curled on a stretcher
like a sleeping snake,

the drunk leaning on a wall,
huffing an unlit cigarette
versus
the pencil-sharpener-blade slits
on a twelve-year-old's wrist.

6.
Someone's shouting orders and though God
has pressed *mute* on the remote,
I know the drill by heart –

pull out the arrest trolley the defibrillator puncture a vein draw blood
secure access no pulse fit the ambubag stick the pads turn off oxygen

stand clear

SHOCK

checkforpulse
the carotid femoral popliteal

stand clear

SHOCK

facesblur

checkforpulse

7.

We wheel her back to the corridor
and drag her down onto the floor.
My colleagues are white dahlia petals
ripped by a centrifugal blast.

8.

Already I am alone shouting for help
but no sound erupts from my mouth.

I shake the mountains of her shoulders,
If you can hear me, open your eyes.

Too little sunlight
has paled our faces.

9.

All the scattered   drug vials

vibrate

and gather
themselves again.

A blue tray flips up
and pulls the ampoules into a neat arrangement.

The collapsed nurse rises
and the tray floats
back to her hands,
warm as steamed plantains.

10.

A pulse ago, I felt the jingle
of the keys she pulled from her pocket.

She drew out fluid
from a vial,

her brown eyes burning out –
I gotta stop this, ya know;
it's my fourth night in a row.
In time, I will retire

and go back to Jamaica.
Check the control with me, will ya?

I puncture a saline bag,
air gurgles up.

11.

Our eyes met from both ends of the corridor. A tacit nod
and she dropped. *Poof!* Gone.

The yellow admission papers in my hands escaped,
flustering at my face into a flight of orioles.

12.

Only God can hear in this chaos
but we learn the drill by heart.

The sounds of rainforest in her jungle-printed bandana
droops from a hook in the staff room.

Grief repeats like a genetic disease,
like a routine drug check.

A shovel tossing dirt
over a sack of bones.

A worker who *can* but *will not*
go back to Jamaica

or the Philippines or España.
Not until Junior has got his diploma,

not until we have nailed a roof on the house
and the pen grunts

with pigs, and the zest of *sinturis*
teems from a once fruitless grove

and we have paid off our parents' grave plots
and our children's –

there – under our forgiving sky
where the wind that rattles our *abaká* forest

is the same wind that pushes an ant
across a puddle,

where the incandescent stalks of *akapulko* flowers wake us
and the weather doesn't come as our perfect pathetic fallacy.

13.
Already I am looking out of the window –
at the landscape etched by horizontal snow.
This red bus leaves now,
it might be the only way to go.

ᜂᜋᜒᜆ

Someone once said: the best way to convince others of your truth
is to wipe away their ᜂᜋᜒᜆ, their *memory*.

No matter how far I've travelled, I can't recall the path back to my
village – the one skirted by a stream and named after five hundred
croaking frogs, said to bring rain and grace the field with rice
stalks.

I only remember our nipa hut – the fruits that thudded onto the
thatched roof and the hands that cracked open a russet shell to find
silver pesos inside.

My grandfather once said: anyone who tells a story is robbed.
Deserted by his father, he made the meat market his home. Each
night, he lay on a stall-table, staring at the stars beyond the ripped
tarp.

Had I listened deeper, I would have heard loose earth blasted by
raindrops. I would have learnt what it was he saw.

~

When the colonisers came, their brightness bleached the scripts
inscribed on our bamboo stems. Our ᜂᜋᜒᜆ was replaced with
their hymn.

I practise writing in Baybayin. Relearning might be the only way
back.

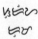

You say our names look like sea waves. The ripple is also the steam of clay-baked *bibingka*, snake trails on the shore, and the wilful undulation of fire.

Even the horizon is curving. Even the lid-handle of my ancestors' burial jar was carved into a boat with a man on the oars and his soul on the bow – to voyage to the afterlife, conveyed by the waves engraved around the vessel's shoulders.

In my version, the boatman and his soul are heading home – the gong of *kulintang* vibrates the marrow in his bones; the seafoam rises with the ballad of benthos and the colours of Tubbataha Reef.

Tahanan ᜆᜈ᜔ means *Home*
Tahan na ᜆ ᜈ᜔ means *Don't cry anymore*

~

Once, an explorer set foot on our land and clothed the *patik* patterns tattooed on my ancestors' torsos. But suppose a strike still stings and each sea wave etched on skin tells a chapter of a slaughter.

Suppose our memory has not been as hollow as bamboo.

My grandfather once said: anyone who tells a story is robbed.
I navigate a blank page with my pen. I will retrieve our ᜇᜋᜒᜆ᜔ and retrace the track back to the clearing that beats with five hundred croaking frogs —

Eponym

Legend says a disciple slipped a clam
into a jade amulet and it persisted to grow –
the Pearl of Lao Tzu. Its lustre spilled over
the valley and peeled the sky with the peal
of Yuqing bells. Perhaps the pendant was flung
in a fit of fury from a delayed enlightenment
or as a gift to calm the Great Ocean's upheaval.
Millennia later, an American called Cobb saved
a *datu*'s child. He was rewarded with a pearl as heavy
as an infant. Resembling the shape of a prophet's
turban, it was then renamed the Pearl of Allah.

I'd like this poem to take you somewhere else
but all I've got is the song of my grandfather
about a fisherman's son whose arms shone
in the bloated glow of the goddess of the moon.
Tides divide at his skull – he swam down to a cathedral
of corals. *Sometime, somewhere,* there was a diver
who hoisted the Pearl of Whoever.
He sat at a table with his wife or – maybe – on his own,
shoulders studded with brine. *Sometime, somewhere,*
there was a fisherman's son who found the world's
largest pearl and we'll never know his name.

The Shaman, The Servant

for my grandfather

And while you were oiling
your hands with *langis ahas*,
whispering incantations
to the hammock of your palm,

                I pushed a needle in
                and the patient fainted;

and while you could erase a headache
with a blow of breath
or draw out poisons by placing
buhay na batô
on a serpent's bite,

                I could only clean
                mould on a wound bed
                with gauze and saline;

and while there was a queue
of villagers at your door
when stars at dawn were rock salts
that buried scarab legs in glass vials,

                a pack outside Lidl
                trailed me on their bicycles,
                shouting, *ching chong;*

and while your house grew with gifts –
a rooster crowing in a *bayong*,
a sack of corn, whiffs of ripe jackfruits,

        a patient woke
        and accused me of stealing
        her job;

and when you stashed
your chants into a chink
in the ceiling beam
and dialled the telephone,

        all I could say was
        I am fine
        and *I've got to go.*

Once, you took in a hawk
and bandaged its wing
with *kakawate* leaves

        and had I known that by August
        the phone would fur with dust,
        I would have pressed the handset
        to my ear, instead of telling you,
        I've got to go,
        it's midnight here.

Ma, the *abaniko* lily has eyes
and the wind has ears of a wild boar –
our neighbours tell me: those who leave
return a *talunan*, a 'loser'.
I didn't believe them. You taught me:
the more fruits a tree bears,
the more men stone it.

Tape Recordings for Mama

The sky is both a praise and a lament –
Ma, remember our neighbour, Luka?
She still sings to the heavens at night.
Every time she claims she owns the *Balatik*
the constellation sinks beneath the horizon.

Ka Celie said Luka had an 'easy-money' job
in Kuwait. Ka Putol said her boss locked her up.
She tallied the days by watching a stream of gold
widen and narrow at her feet. She returned
without any jewels apart from anklet-thick scars.

Take care, Ma. Don't worry about us here.

Tape Recordings for Mama

Repairing English

You cautioned me against using *like* –
told me the stink of shrimp paste was sickening, like

ridiculous: What is ridiculous? My true being
or my sentences tripping over *likes*?

I want to find meaning, so I Google *like*
and learn it is an *extensible* word; then I Google

extensible. A sofa bed clacks wide – and sinks
with the bulk of a man who anticipates the likelihood

of grief. His wife's bluing lips. When I say I don't like
the cold, I don't mean the snowstorm seen from this floor

of a hospital window – the whirr of a whiteout, godlike.
I think of my Nanay Lola who couldn't afford dialysis

everytime I say getting sick in my country is like
suicide. On a jeepney to Manila, she yanked out a butterfly

knife, and turned it on a man who was pulling her purse.
When I say I don't like the cold, I only miss the likes

of our summer – when our ground flares with ginger lilies,
but whenever I close my eyes, I see Nanay Lola

and the man whose blood was gushing out of his waist
like Nanay Lola had drilled a faucet into it and left it open.

Mastering English

In the UK, when they say the *sky* is not working, they mean:
☐ God is too high to hear your prayers
☐ The television channel

The phrase *a drop in the ocean* indicates:
☐ Very little amount in comparison to what is expected or needed
☐ All the migrants who mysteriously vanished at sea

An arm and a leg is:
☐ The constellation Marara, deity of rainclouds, seen from the porch where your colleague-housemate used to sit with her younger brother
☐ What she says as she turns off her heater

What does *I'm just popping out* mean?
☐ A man rattling a bolted door, adamant to fetch his daughter from school, even if his daughter has already had daughters of her own
☐ Your lie when you left your child to work in another country

If the charge nurse declares, *It's neither here nor there*, you must understand it as:
☐ something unimportant or irrelevant
☐ an opportunity to ask, 'Where is it, then?'

Anosmia

At first, it is uncomfortable,
and you must distract yourself,
burrow your nose through the half-
opened foil lid of a Fortisip, or gaze
at a square of sky through the window.

Soon, you get used to it: routinely part
your legs for the nurse with bronzed
skin, whose look you can never read:
Has she got used to the stench
of solitude? Is she just pretending?

You learn about anosmia and kindness.
You stop saying 'Sorry, how embarrassing.'
You learn the weight of her touch,
the way a wipe glides down your groin
and the slight push of her palm on your hip.

You roll onto your side, and don't fear
falling off. You memorise the stories
of her town – the cow rides, and the man
who put a plumeria behind her ear,
her breath warming the end of your spine.

Only Distance

When all the stars are out, she returns
to this tropical wind, to the constellation

of moles on his shoulder, his second-hand clothes.
He slices mangoes and lays them on a banana leaf.

She's with him – the child now half a foot taller
than her. A cigarette ember penetrates the dark –

if only ash would fall and stop mid-air.
His cough shakes the branches of his lungs,

siniguelas and *salagubang* thump to the ground –
those nights they cut through cane fields, bathed

in forest fireflies. He says, *Smoking kills*
but only distance can break the heart.

The day she leaves for her foreign home,
she embraces the weight of the plane taking off

but when the seatbelt light pings, she imagines
the year from now – the hut by the sea

and the *kanin* grains bubbling in a bamboo stem
over a campfire. She can see his finger sliding into

the head of a fish, hooking the gills out. His time-
conscious smile, the brilliance of salt-sprinkling.

The Wait

'Every pot has a matching lid.' – TAGALOG PROVERB

I'd like to incise you the way a cook skins cod,
separating the pure meat with one sure slice.

The boundary between us is as thin
as the acidic air. You say it's *just a piece*

of paper. What more could we want?
Yes, there are worse things than words –

I am a tendril that stretches towards sunlight.
You are an animal hooked by the mouth.

We are fish and chips
in a Styrofoam tray,

the night a sour tang and the breeze
runs through my fingers. Don't be mad

if I told you I used to wait at an *isawan*
in front of my old school – flashing potential

Prince Charmings a smile. Come, I'll take you
to an *isawan* where Ka Celie pulled florets

of intestines out of a chicken tail slit. The stall
has graduated to a ramshackle restaurant,

now run by Ka Celie's son.
On a table, there is a plaque that reads:

47

Don't think about the wait,
what's important is
it will come.

Ma, *kamusta na?*
The morning arrived
as a grown *haribon*'s shadow
stitching the length of a jungle's river.

Before dusk, the eagle
descends back to its nest.
I squint at the brightness
of its widespread underwings.

Tape Recordings for Mama

Checkmate

My father said, *Take advantage*
of the position of your pieces.

Do you think a crab spider
camouflages itself on a petal
just to fit in?

Checkmate in four moves.

Suppose my life in the UK
is not unplanned, and this time

God is giving me a better chance.
I pacify the cries of an old woman
for her long-cremated mother

with Lorazepam in a spoonful of yogurt.

No move is unplanned.
We walk together, palm to palm,

down *Jon Speelman Street* corridor.
We sit on a waiting bench,
a plastic robin perched

on a plastic Bus Stop sign.

She strokes my face and tells me
I look as young as the queen.

My father said, *No move is unplanned.*
Perhaps here I have a better chance.
I am not a queen, but a pawn

inching to the other side.

Respecting the Nunò

My grandfather warns:
    If I twist a bud off a twig without the *nunò*'s consent,
        my feet will bulge like an elephant's.
    If I sweep at night, luck will bleed out of my life.
    If I crane my neck, ululating like a mournful soul,
        coins will drop soundlessly to the ground.
    If I chop a tree's bough or crush an ant mound,
        my hands will crumble into maggots.
    At a wake, the youngest family member must jump
over the corpse, otherwise – I forget the consequence.
    When my elderly patient sleeps my steps must land
as light as paper so the blank *next of kin* box will not echo
        an avalanche. Alone on Christmas Eve,
his scalp smoulders with the reflection of gold-foil garlands.
    It was drought when I last saw my grandfather doused
in a shaft of sunrise – blue steam rises from his cup.
    He called to me, *Kape tayo. Come, sit with me.* I sit
by my patient's bedside and find a fraction of what I've lost.

A nunò is a dwarf-like spirit who lives in an anthill, but also means
'grandparent' in Tagalog.

For the Dance Festival

You clothe me
in a frock made of reeds,
dyed in soaked annatto seeds.
This is the colour of our tribe.
You say, *Tingnan mo*
ang mundo – Look at the world
as you brush back my hair
and hold it in place
with a headdress –
panicles of tiger grass
fanned around my skull.

I want to be fair skinned
like an alabaster goddess,
like Romblon marble.
But your calloused fingers smear
crushed charcoal on my face.
Only the whites of my eyes
and the ant-red tint of my lips
recall a forgotten tradition.
Your hand beckons:
Maffick down the road,
let loose the Ati-atihan in you.

Ma, what did you wear at your prom?
Outside San Sebastian, I saw a dress
sequined with streaks of twilight.
Please buy it for me, Ma.

Ma, *kamusta na?* The morning
came forth in a torn drape
with news about a London
bus bombing. Come home, Ma.

Please come home
and buy that dress for me, Ma.

———————————————

Tape Recordings for Mama

A Manananggal Replies to a Child

The Storyteller gathered you
with the village children every night –
his marble floor oiled by moonlight.

He claimed I crashed onto his roof,
pierced it with my tongue that elongated
down towards his sleeping son.

Since then, you've hung garlic bundles
above the doorway, kept a packet
of rock salt to keep me at bay.

But a secret unfolds into a pair of wings –
my stomach muscles tear apart,
each tendon snaps, seethes like sulphur.

I am halved in order to be whole –
I rebuild by leaving
everything I love.

I soar – my frayed skin drips blood
onto the shadowed streets,
onto the plaza where children sleep.

My blood clatters and fills
the can of a man slumped at an *eskinita* –
his left eye rotting with a clump of flies.

In a city cremated by its residual light,
would you not wish to leave your body?
Child, would you not take flight?

Aren't women more beautiful
when they scab into beasts?
Aren't mothers more lamentable

when they don't die but leave? –
to glide over newer cities where rooftops
in their kamacite-glint, make you believe

in houses with windows that flicker
in the glow of new *lampara*,
where a banquet table blisters

with cakes and cherry gelatins
and every bed has sheets
warm as skin.

I am halved in order to be whole –
I rebuild by leaving
everything I love.

The Storyteller didn't warn you
that one day you could be
the one scavenging

for thrown-away meat,
your father the man
with an empty can at his feet.

No thumb tracing pearl rosaries, no salt,
no garlic dangling at the threshold
can deter me. In the jungle

of my ribcage
a heart flares – about to rip
the night into songs.

Let the town enumerate my faults
and hunt down my lower half; my intestines
pulverise in the shine of thrown salt

and I risk not finding my way back.
In another life I'm just another mother,
praying we make it to daybreak –

my fingertips dipped in *banal na tubig*
in a clam poised on a stone angel's palm.
My collarbones sparkle with a bead

necklace from you, my child.
For now, my blood floods the cities
that pass through me, my shoulder blades

protrude and fracture into an expanse
of bat-like wings. One day you'll see
a flock of women severed by the waist

swarm around me –
churning with the fury
of typhoons. Hear the riot of our wings

and learn, my child – mothers
are *manananggal*, meshing the sky
that is always the colour of shredded flesh.

relearning

soon i will remember   the man in a wicker hat
       he picked the biggest *balot* from the nest
                 of steaming towels   in his basket

and again   yesterday will crack
at the corner of a table   i will un-shell the egg's rounded tip   and sip the broth
before hunting for the chick's head   suave with black feathers   the tiny beak
       the soft skull   will crumble
                     in my mouth

i will learn again   how my mother laughs
      after three eye surgeries   how she tells me
i'm still beautiful   though i have a cloud for a face

once   she placed   a pig's trotter   with a slit skin   beside a suture pack
     in front of a student nurse   whose bones i once lived in
they practised stitching wounds   throughout the plasticity of the night

i will sleep again   convinced there's nothing to worry
      about how distance   distorts the hail of a *balot* vendor
      or the nights when lizards drop onto my bed
or the patient   whose own mother   could not legally identify
until the police reconstructed   his broken face
tomorrow   will bring the music of broomsticks   against the soil
     guava leaves snapping   on fire

one day   i will uncover my mouth
and the atavistic *balot*   will be appetising again
i will get a glimpse   of the mirror ghost   on a thunderous night
   and shatter   in laughter again
      i will trust   and play chess
       against myself again

Kayumanggi

Remember the myth – the night you lifted your arm
to the light, adoring the *kayumanggi*-gleam of your skin –

how God moulded people from clay. He was hasty once,
not firing the first clump of clay-men long enough,

then careless for burning the next batch. Turn your back
on the brash-blinking tarmac, on the next-door lad

on a narra ladder who festoons festive lights, and yells
with a lancet-sharp snigger, *Ang itim! You're ugly!*

If a shadow of a teak tree spills and pins you at your feet,
remember darkness is neither the absence of light

nor the abundance of shades. Might as well let bygones
be bygones – the bucket that bobbed in a brimming tub

and you, the ugly duckling who scrubbed and scrubbed.
Go ahead – trail that next-door boy and mock his body

glazed in sewage sludge after a ladder fall. Soon,
a whistle pulls you to a bench. The breeze persuades

a hanging lantern. Memorise your mother's story
of God's endurance, and learn that on his third try

he gaped at the last batch of clay people
and was satisfied.

Ode to a Pot Noodle

Salt-sharp, *umami*-hint of steam
seeps from the unfastened lid.

A cluster of noodles softens in a pot,
a body unstiffens in its new climate.

You sustain me during break, a breath
before an emergency bell tears a wall.

Oh, I will pedestal you on the counter
in the limelight of this lonely bulb,

this fast-paced night, this instant life.
A radiator click-clacks at the corner

where I find a vapour of my grandfather in his
arthritic dance, stirring something at the stove.

Garlics are chopped, peppercorns are cracked,
and the shadows of my *pamilya* ripple at the *mesa*.

I smile at their unflavoured conversations,
how they slurp marrow from shanks of *bulalô* bones,

spoon-scrape the meat from the carapaces of crabs.
How everyone evaporates when the kettle snaps.

And yes, this should have been an ode to you.
Forgive me, forgive me.

Group Portrait at the Stopover

'take a walk / over the sharp stones / then come back'
– NERUDA

I.

Elbow to elbow on waiting chairs.
We rummage through our luggage for treasures
and out flitter sunbirds. I lift the 24 carat
radiance of butter fudge. Take this. *Sige na,*
and I will accept your focaccia and basbousa.

II.

Manong, tell me your story until the whole terminal
smells of petrol and rust. Salt-soaked tanker.
The skyscraper-tide that almost sank your ship
is now the wind beating the viewing glass.
Remember the afternoons that could burn
a dragonfly, the oil-stickiness of your wife's lips,
and the baby you left one night, who by the morning
of your return, had turned into a man with a beard.

III.

Manang, you keep glancing at me. For a moment
I thought the burn mark on your cheek
was a spotted moth wing. I am listening. Whisper
of the days you must dab garlic on your wrists,
smear grease on your neck, so *Sir* won't grab.
Speak of the years you spent sleeping on floors –
beside potatoes and pickle jars, and the day
you learned how to arrange flowers for visitors,

fill the vases with faithful water, admire the petals
whose edges are like saw teeth.

IV.

Manong, Manang, take these, and I will tell you
how I pull out (with five colleagues) a bariatric man
from the driver's seat and start chest compressions
in the hospital car park. I will take you there –
between rushing to A&E and the doctor yelling:
                                    Jump on him!
Jump there with me – on top of the stretcher, the man
between your legs, your hands pumping his heart.
Do not fear the clatter of wheels, the bumps
and slopes in corridors. It is only turbulence.

V.

Let these Duty Free bags distract our loved ones
from the scars on our feet. *Tara na*, let's not think,
for now, of the next generation that will meet at this gate,
the same old stories that will hum out of younger mouths.
Let's go home – to our elders' kitchens
where tapioca pearls soften in the choir of casseroles.

Para sa mga batang naiwan
   or For the children left behind

May there be a portion of sky
for those who sleep tentless in the field,
for those who climb trees, pretending
the fruits in their pockets are grenades,
shouting back at the fang of lightning in the sky.

Antiemetic for Homesickness

A day will come when you won't miss
the country *na nagluwal sa 'yo.*
You'll walk on gritted streets, light snow
shawling you like a mother's warmth.

A vertigo of distant lights will not deceive you.
Bury all the kisses of yesterday in the fold
of your handkerchief – the illuminated
star-shaped lanterns, the *tansan* tambourines.

But keep the afternoon your father sold his buffalo
to rent a jeepney to take you to the airport,
the driver who spat out phlegm with the trajectory
of a grasshopper that lands on the ground.

Keep the list you wrote the night before you left –
a promise to not return till you become *somebody.*
Keep the cassette tapes – your children's voices
shrill as the edges of winter stars.

Keep the booklet of *Our Lady of Perpetual Help*
in your uniform pocket, powder blue
like her robe. Say the rosary,
feel each *kamagong* bead.

Rest on a pillow to sense the rise
and fall of your husband's chest. Listen
to Tagalog songs, they will help you sleep
through the cold scratches of December.

Here is the tea-stained smile of a *kababayan*
who invites you to a party. Go –
no matter how heavy the day has been
and how many corpses you have carried within.

Enjoy the homecooked *pansit guisado*,
the roasted pig's head, the blood-red apple
in its mouth. A day will come
when you won't need an antiemetic

for homesickness. You will accept
the patient's relative who always buzzes
for a commode, the search for the missing boot
of an A&E habitué – the village drunk.

You will learn to heal the wounds
of their lives and the wounds of yours.
Love even the smoke
of a Brummie accent on your face.

So, here is the karaoke mic –
sing your soul out until there's El Niño
in your throat, and you can drink
all the rain of Wolverhampton.

A Boodle Fight of Words and Terminologies

abaká: a species of banana tree endemic to the Philippines, whose fibres are harvested to make textiles and clothes.

Ang itim: can be literally translated as 'so dark'.

Ati-atihan: a dance festival celebrated in Aklan, Philippines. It includes tribal street dances, and the use of indigenous costumes and weapons.

banal na tubig: holy water.

bayong: a bag made of woven, dried *buri* leaves.

bulalô: a type of beef shank soup popular in the province of Batangas.

bibingka: baked rice cake.

buhay na batô: a 'living stone', believed to heal or draw out poisons from dog or snake bites.

capiz: windowpane oyster, mostly found in the eponymous province of Capiz.

dalanghita: a small fruit-bearing tree largely cultivated in Batangas. In folkloric medicine, the oil from its rind is believed to relieve ache and inflammation.

datu: title of a chieftain ruler in the Middle and Southern Philippines.

El Niño: a climate cycle that occurs in the tropical Pacific Ocean. In the Philippines, this climate marks the beginning of severe drought.

eskinita: an unlit alleyway.

isawan: a side-walk stall that sells skewered chicken intestines, heads, feet, pork liver, and other light snacks.

kababayan: a term of endearment to a fellow Filipino migrant; literally 'townmate' or 'fellow country man'.

kamagong: a hardwood of the *kamagong* tree, native to the Philippines.

kamias: a fruit from bilimbi tree, used as a souring agent for dishes.

kamote: a type of sweet potato.

Kamusta na?: 'How have you been?'

kanin: rice.

kangkong: water spinach; mostly found in the backyards of Filipino households.

kulintang: an ancient musical instrument made of small horizontally laid gongs.

langis-ahas: snake oil.

lolo: grandfather.

lomi: a type of thick egg noodle-soup, a speciality dish of Batangas province.

makopa: java apple.

manananggal: a legendary creature in Philippine folktale. She is an ordinary woman by day but by night she severs herself in half and transforms into a winged monster.

na nagluwal sa 'yo: can be literally translated as 'who gave birth to you'.

Noche Buena: a traditional meal shared by Filipino families during Christmas Eve.

pansit guisado: a type of stir-fried noodles, a fusion of Chinese and Spanish influence.

patik: intricate patterns tattooed on native Visayan people, signifying strength and beauty.

pavo: peacock.

sabong: a cockfight, considered as a pastime in the Philippines.

salagubang: June bug, found in the foliage of trees.

sampaguita: white jasmines.

Simbang Gabi: a Catholic mass attended in the late hours of Christmas Eve.

siniguelas: also known as Spanish plum.

tagay: a term for the penchant to drink together from the same glass passed around in a circle among the drinkers.

tansan: pressed bottle caps.
Wala kang kwenta: translates as 'You're useless'.

Notes

'**Half-empty**': The poem's epigraph is taken from a remark made by Prince Philip to a Filipino nurse at his visit at Luton and Dunstable University Hospital (*Evening Standard*, 2013).

'**Names**': The poem's epigraph is from *An Open Letter to Filipino Artists* by Emmanuel Lacaba (1976).

'**The Making of a Smuggler**': is after Zilka Joseph's 'The Rice Fields'.

'**Way Back Home**': The poem's epigraph is from *Slow Chrysanthemums: Classical Korean Poems in Chinese* (Anvil Press, 1987).

'**Notes inside a Balikbayan Box**': OFWs (overseas Filipino workers) spend a fraction of their monthly wages on small gifts to put inside a 'Balikbayan box'. Once full, they send the box to their loved ones in the Philippines. Thus, 'Balikbayan box' translates as 'repatriate box'.

'**To Die a Little**': The poem references the title of Randy VanWarmer's song, 'Just When I Needed You Most', a song often played by our neighbourhood *mang-iinom* (drinkers) and one of the first English songs that reminded me of my mother when she was away.

'**At the Other End of the Bridge**': Traditionally in the Philippines, when someone leaves her village, her lover sends her off by watching her cross the bridge that connects their village to the next. On her return, the lover is at the other end of the bridge waiting. Thus, in Filipino culture, bridges symbolise both connection and separation.

'**Tagay! [Drinking Lambanog with my Filipino Colleagues]**': It is part of OFW culture to create a community to support each other while they are away from home. This poem is in the *tagay* form, a drinking song in Philippine folk poetry.

'**Nature Morte aux Tulipes**': In early 2018, Joanna Demafelis, an OFW in Kuwait, was found mutilated in her employer's freezer. This ekphrasis-sonnet is for her and for every exile-by-employment whose leaving poses great risks to their lives.

'[   ]': In 2016, a red bus was used to campaign for Brexit, suggesting the vote to leave would help fund the NHS. 65,000 NHS staff in England are EU Nationals while Filipinos are the third most common nationality of NHS Staff (Parliament UK, 2019).

This poem is for every migrant worker in the NHS whose strength emanates from their dream of a better life for their families back home, and especially for all my comrades who have risked their own welfare in service to the British public.

'ᜄᜒᜈᜒᜆ' (**Gunita**): This poem uses Baybayin, an ancient script of the Tagalog people that is no longer used today. The script in this poem is in its indigenous version and not to be confused with the version modified by the Spaniards to represent modern sounds.

'**Eponym**': Until 2016, The Pearl of Lao Tzu or The Pearl of Allah, found in Palawan Philippines, was once regarded as the world's largest known pearl. The new title holder was also found in the seas of Palawan.

'Tape Recordings for Mama': the last two lines on page 41 reference a Tagalog proverb.

'A Manananggal Replies to a Child': This poem takes the form of *uyayi*, or cradle song. In Philippine folk poetry, *uyayi* poems are sung not only as lullabies, they are also a device in which mothers can communicate the hardships of life to their children.

'Kayumanggi': In Tagalog mythology, clay people who were fired too briefly had the lightest skin (mestizo/mestiza), clay people who were fired for too long had the darkest shade (aeta/katutubo), and the last clay people were fired 'just right', thus, getting the shade of kayumanggi.

'Group Portrait at the Stopover': The poem's epigraph is taken from *Then Come Back: The Lost Neruda*, translated by Forrest Gander (Copper Canyon Press, 2016).

Acknowledgements

Thank you po, Lord.

Thank you mother, for showing me what real strength is and for teaching me the value of believing in life, especially if it takes us to difficult places. Thank you father, for teaching me best in silence, a chess board between us. Thank you, my grandparents, for teaching me that in order to preserve a memory, we must be willing to share it. Thank you, my uncles, aunties, and our neighbourhood drunkards for first teaching me the beauty of music through your *gitara* and tipsy songs.

Thank you to the editors of the following magazines where some of these poems appeared in their earlier stages: *Poetry Review*, *The Rialto*, *Ambit*, *Oxford Poetry*, *Magma*, *Smoke* and *The Good Journal*. Some of the poems in this collection also appeared in *Midnight Listening* (Jerwood/Arvon Anthology 2018) and *Primers Volume 3* (Nine Arches Press/ The Poetry School). 'Patis' first appeared in my pamphlet, *Rice & Rain* (V Press, 2017). 'A Manananggal Replies to a Child' first appeared on Bedtime Stories for the End of the World podcast. 'The Making of a Smuggler' received commendation in Battered Moons Poetry Competition 2017. 'Way Back Home' won the Creative Future Literary Award 2017. 'Antiemetic for Homesickness' is one of the poems joint-awarded the Manchester Poetry Prize 2017. 'Names' won the Poetry London Clore Prize 2018. 'To Die a Little' received second prize in the Oxford Brookes Poetry Competition EAL Category 2019.

Thank you Parisa and my Chatto family, for trusting me. Thank you to the following organisations who moulded me into the artist I am now: Writing West Midlands, Jerwood/

Arvon Mentoring Programme, Primers 3 of Nine Arches Press and The Poetry School, and Silliman University National Writers Workshop.

I would not be able to write these poems if it weren't for the kind support of Arts Council England's Developing Your Creative Practice grant, Hosking Houses and Shakespeare Birthplace Trust, and The Society of Author's The Author's Foundation award.

A shot of coconut wine to my mentors whose influence will always be a part of me:

Pascale Petit (and Jerwood/Arvon), thank you for the wisdom and the laughter. You taught me the importance of giving my poem a heart that illuminates.

Ahren Warner (and Creative Future Literary Award in partnership with The Literary Consultancy), thank you for teaching me the power of perseverance and line breaks, and for showing me how to interrogate the mind of my poems.

Marjorie Evasco (and Developing Your Creative Practice of Arts Council England), thank you for guiding me on my way home and for always reminding me that no matter how adorned a cart is, it cannot move by itself.

Thanks also to these wonderful souls who encouraged and helped me along the way: Jonathan, Liz and our Birmingham workshop group, Jane, Hannah, Stuart, Alice, Yvonne, Seraphima, Ron, Raymond, Troy, Julie, Natalie, Dan, Kostya, and Cynthia. Thanks also to Filip + Inna for support.

To my love, Suriya, and to our two baby dogs, Tia and Jiraiya, thank you.

Someone told me once that a poet is a pilgrim and the journey is hard on the spirit. Everyone, *maraming salamat*, thank you, for being there with me.

And thank you, dear reader, for truly listening.